GU00982955

CBD OIL
FOR PAIN RELIEF

Your Complete Guide to CBD Oil for Natural
and Effective Pain Relief without Medications

Published by the Fruitful Mind LTD.
www.thefruitfulmind.com

DISCLAIMER

INTRODUCTION

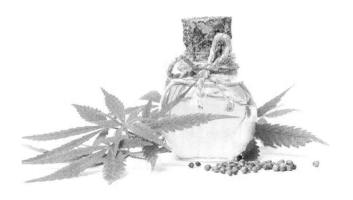

So often, we're told to "just deal with it." We're told to deal with the pain, the anxiety, the depression of our everyday lives—popping the occasional pill just to get through. This leads to a poor quality of life. It leads to us growing sicker and fatter and more fatigued, fighting our bodies' very real processes and neural alert systems. Each and every day, we fall further away from our bodies' needs, from natural, healing properties of plants and foods, until we inevitably crash in a pit of pain and despair.

And we do it because we're not told there's another option.

Rather than work against the pain, using ibuprofen, or even more serious medications, it's essential to find a more natural healing process. And with the advancements in our understanding of CBD oil in the previous few decades, there's no legitimate reason we shouldn't be utilizing its incredible properties for healing, each and every day. That's especially if you're debilitated by pain, whether that pain is chronic or just momentary. That's also if you're dealing with depression and anxiety associated with the pain and suffering, as CBD oil has been linked to enhancing cognitive abilities as well.

In fact, CBD oil has been linked to healing many different ailments, including fibromyalgia, which is a kind of pain that seems to sizzle throughout the entire body (in fact, fibromyalgia was only recently regarded as a "real" illness two decades ago—and could be linked to stress and anxiety). CBD oil has been known to heal chronic pain, which is the kind of pain that lingers after twelve weeks or more.

Also, CBD oil has been studied extensively as a way to fight the inflammation found in rheumatoid arthritis. And in some cases CBD oil has even been shown to decrease the rapid advancement of rheumatoid arthritis, meaning that you can actually buck back against a "death sentence" of sorts and live a more normal life.

Furthermore, for those suffering with multiple sclerosis, who are debilitated, experiencing spasms and spastic motions, CBD oil has been proven to decrease this at an incredible rate. The testimonials are incredible, but the results are better.

In this book, we discuss what CBD oil is: how it affects your body, its very, very few side effects, its legality, and how it can work, starting today, to heal you. We discuss specific studies that have been linked to the various aches and pains, and then we dive into the gritty mathematical details of just how much you should be taking, based on your weight and how much pain you're experiencing. This is a confusing new world— one that's unnecessarily linked to "druggies" and the fringe of the law. Come over to the "dark side" of using plants and natural elements to heal yourself.

CBD oil is a relatively new field, which means that new research is coming out all the time, as are new brands, new ways of taking it, and new ways of healing yourself naturally. Armed with this book, you can find answers to what seemed like a sentence to continued pain. You can find relief.

TABLE OF CONTENTS

CHAPTER 1:

CBD Oil for Pain Relief: What is it, and how does it work?

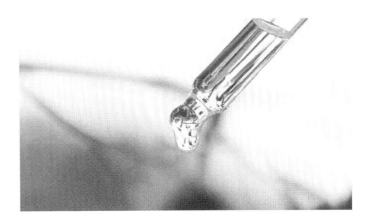

CBD oil, otherwise known by its longer name, cannabidiol, is one of over sixty of the compounds found in the cannabis—or marijuana plant. Immediately, this gives it a bad name throughout much of the world (although it's completely legal). Unlike its brothers, tetrahydrocannabinol, or THC, or other cannabidiol compounds, CBD oil actually doesn't create the "high" usually associated with marijuana. Rather, it's used for medical purposes, and exhibits an incredibly different reaction in the brain and body.

CBD Oil: Not From Your Typical Hemp Plant

Generally speaking, the CBD oil that we use for medical purposes is taken from a plant that's bred industrially, meaning that it isn't the "natural hemp" that's generally used for THC and marijuana smoking. After extracting the CBD compound, marijuana makers generally mix it with an oil, and then term it "CBD oil." It's taken in a variety of ways, including via pill, orally, via a spray, or topically. We'll discuss the many different ways (and what's best for you based on your current pain problems) in a later chapter.

A Brief History of CBD Oil

CBD cannabis has been utilized for pain relief for several hundred years. Back in the 1800s, for example, Queen Victoria of England utilized CBD oil to treat her cramps during her period, and she did this frequently, relying on it as her singular treatment. After that, however, people turned away from CBD oil, until, in the 1980s, studies showed that CBD could hold answers for things like anxiety, nausea, and pain relief.

Unfortunately for us, these studies didn't get much press until a decade later, in the '90s.

This occurred when an individual named Geoffrey Guy, one of the founders of a company called GW Pharmaceuticals in England, began to extract cannabis for medicinal purposes. From the research conducted during this time, it became apparent that CBD decreased seizures and anxiety in trials, which forced the rest of the world to pay attention. By the time 2009 hit—over ten years after that, a lab in Oakland, California had begun cultivating strains of cannabis that contained more CBD than THC—which was essential to decrease the psychoactive properties and give it complete medicinal benefits.

After this, the public began to take notice as well, especially as CBD oil began to affect the lives of people across the world. Namely, a family in Montana began to utilize CBD oil for their baby son, who had brain cancer. According to the baby's doctor, the baby's tumor was inoperable, and it was getting worse and worse all the time. This was even after thirty rounds of radiation, heavy morphine, and other medicines which basically knocked the baby out with side effects.

The baby's father turned to CBD oil, not knowing what else to do. After a first administration of high concentration CBD oil, the baby's tumor had actually shrunk. The baby lived for another two years after that, despite having had a pretty immediate death sentence. Most notably, the baby actually passed away after Montana made it more difficult for the family to purchase the CBD oil.

Other stories involving depression, anxiety, tumors, pain, seizures, arthritis, and countless other ailments are prolific and far-reaching. CBD oil has made a dramatic impact on the past ten years, during a time when stress and illnesses are at an all-time high. Turning away from lab-made medicines could be the key to get us back to our natural roots. It could be the key to greater health.

The Difference between Hemp Oil and Cannabis Oil

When looking to self-medicate and treat your bodily pain, it's important to not mix up hemp oil and cannabis oil. It can be an easy mistake to make, given the fact that they both are derived from similar plants—and are often called the same thing, by accident. Especially if you go to the wrong online forums (there's a LOT of misinformation out there).

CBD oil and hemp oil both come from the same plant genus, called Cannabis. But within that genus are three different species of plants, entitled the indica, the sativa, and the ruderalis. The strains from cannabis sativa and cannabis indica are generally found at your local marijuana dispensary (if you come from some of the western states, or other areas where marijuana is legal). The cannabis ruderalis, however, is generally grown in the wild and is known to be lower in THC, or the compound that makes you high.

Both CBD oil and hemp oil are generally denied from cannabis sativa. However, hemp oil and CBD oil are derived from different strains of the cannabis sativa. The strains are made in different ways to create different highs or aromas or CBD counts or THC counts.

Hemp oil is taken from the seeds of the hemp plant. This is similar to olives, coconuts, or other seeds—all of which we use for their medicinal and nutritional properties. Hemp oil is used much the same and is often turned to for recipes and salad dressings.

CBD oil, on the other hand, is made from the leaves, flowers and plant stalks of the plant, meaning that it has a completely different makeup.

Neither the hemp oil nor the CBD oil are used to get that famous THC "high." However, only CBD oil can be utilized for medicinal purposes or pain relief, while hemp oil has other uses. In fact, both hemp oil and CBD oil have a THC concentration of 0.3% or lower, which isn't a concentration that you can derive a high from.

The Endocannabinoid System and CBD Oil

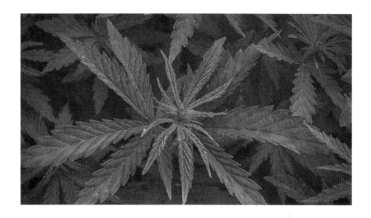

As mentioned, your body reacts differently to THC, or the compound found in marijuana, than it does to the compounds in CBD oil, despite them both being taken from the same plant.

What's the reason for this difference in how your body reacts to CBD oil versus THC?

CBD oil simply doesn't fill the same receptors in the brain. Essentially, the human body has a system called the "endocannabinoid system," which sends and receives signals that it takes from any imbibed, smoked, or even cannabinoids that your body creates itself. This endocannabinoid system regulates things in your body such as what pain you experience, your immune system, your appetite, your sexual drive, and even just how much you sleep. It's heavily linked to your circadian rhythm, for example, ensuring that you sleep during the nighttime and stay awake during the day (at least, it's supposed to—but in our strange, new-era lifestyles, these hormones are often wonky, leading to things like insomnia and depression. That's what CBD oil can cure).

CBD oil, unlike THC, creates a very complex system of reactions in your endocannabinoid system. While THC activates the "pleasure" receptors in your brain making food taste better and your jokes funnier, CBD oil acts in a way that allows your body to utilize its endocannbinoids in a better and more economical way.

Perhaps most importantly, for the sake of this book, we'll be focusing on the fact that CBD oil can affect the way you experience pain. For example, when taken, CBD oil stops the body from absorbing something called anandamide. When you have more anandamide in your bloodstream and body, you can reduce the amount of pain you feel.

Furthermore, CBD oil may decrease the amount of inflammation that affects your greater nervous system, including your brain. This could alleviate several types of pain, and even sleepless nights associated with insomnia.

Overall known uses of CBD oil include the following:

1. Protection of your neural pathways
2. Decrease in inflammation
3. Decrease in signs of depression
4. Decrease in anxiety
5. Fight the growth of some tumors
6. Decrease risk of seizures and epilepsy
7. Antioxidant
8. Decrease in levels of psychosis
9. Decrease in signs of anorexia
10. Better sleep
11. Fights pain
12. Fights nausea
13. Decrease in menstrual pain
14. Decreases risk of diabetes
15. Boosts your heart health

Look to the following chapters to learn the legality of CBD oil, how it can heal your neck and back pain, how it can heal your fibromyalgia, how to fight multiple sclerosis, how to dose, and how to take it. Your body and mind are waiting for relief.

CHAPTER 2:
Is CBD Oil Legal? Reading Between the Legal Lines

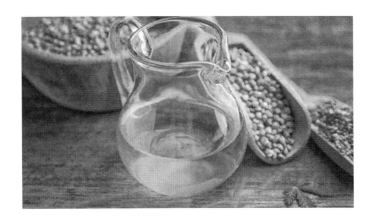

CBD oil is taken from the same plant as THC, the compound that makes up marijuana. Cannabis is generally regulated throughout much of the world, and most of the United States. However, due to the fact that CBD oil is medicinal in nature, and not used for recreational purposes, it's actually legal in all 50 states: as long as we follow a few restrictions.

Taking CBD oil for medicinal purposes is one hundred percent legal, as long as the CBD oil products come from an industrial hemp plant. When it's taken from just a regular hemp plant, and not derived professionally, the THC content of the oil is probably too high for medicinal purposes.

According to the DEA, or the Drug Enforcement Agency, CBD products which are derived from industrial hemp are completely and totally legal within the American states, as long as they have less than a 0.3% level of THC.

How To Know Your CBD Oil is Genuine and Legal

The CBD oil is a tricky one, as many people may be looking to rip you off. It's difficult to get CBD oil without THC: requiring a complex series of processes, which most people cannot possibly do at home. This puts many companies in the position of overstating their product, even as they cut corners and potentially even give you CBD oil with over the legal limit of THC: meaning it's over 0.3% in potency, and making your medicinal foray into the industry completely illegal.

Therefore, it's best to go with one of the brands we'll discuss in a later chapter, and to always ensure that you're calculating how many milligrams of CBD is in the bottle you purchase. We'll talk about not getting ripped off by dealers in a later chapter.

Midwest Confusion: CBD Oil Raids and Arrests

In the past year, Midwesterners, especially, have taken to CBD oil to search for healing and relief, due to the fact that medicinal marijuana isn't available to them (as it is in more of the western states, including Colorado and California). However, most notably, Indiana governor Eric Holcomb threatened CBD oil retailers that they must remove CBD oil from their shelves, which shows that the legality of these things is often confused even amongst the higher-ups in government.

Furthermore, another Indiana man was recently charged with marijuana possession for having CBD oil in his car. An outlet researching the CBD oil that was found in his car calculated that the oil had zero percent of THC—well below the legal limit, meaning that the man's charge was completely against the law.

In order to stay within the bounds of the law, ensure you purchase your CBD oil from a well-documented, legal source, which we'll outline in a later chapter. Make sure that it's always below 0.3% THC, and that it's derived from an industrial hemp plant. Don't mess around with the legality of this CBD oil world, as it's still iffy on many sides—with even higher-ups, like the Indiana government, not quite sure what's right and what's wrong.

CHAPTER 3:
Neck or Back Pain and CBD Oil

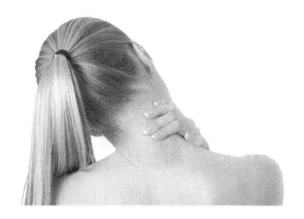

Back and neck pain is a plague on millions of people around the world. The treatments that are available for neck and back pain are simple at best, and can only heal so much. And most of the medications that you can take for neck and back pain actually cause damage to other bodily organs, meaning that you're putting a band-aide on one problem while pouring acid over another problem.

In many cases, people with neck and back pain seek out surgery for relief, when things like medications and neuropathy don't work out. This can be costly and can lead to further complications. After all: any time you go under the knife, you leave yourself open to countless predicaments. Surgery mistakes do happen.

However, know that CBD oil is an option for neck and back pain.

What Normally Causes Back or Neck Pain?

You've probably seen photographs of spines before. The spine is made up of a series of discs, which are made up of cartilage. The cartilage is meant to ensure that the shock of walking, running, and living doesn't wear on the bones. However, as you age, the cartilage discs begin to decay, which causes back and neck pain on a deep level, in your bones.

Usually, this decay is caused by several factors, including a lack of oxygen, a lack of hydration and water, poor diet, and just general inflammation from everyday life.

According to the Medicine of the National Academies, over one hundred million Americans are currently living with this back and neck pain. And generally speaking, these one hundred million Americans are treated with anti-inflammatory drugs, otherwise known as NSAIDS. These drugs are probably pretty familiar to you. They include ibuprofen, which is just pain relief, or even valium, which allows your muscles to relax. And incredibly, ibuprofen is actually said to be the most effective treatment for back pain—even though it can often lead to stomach ulcers, constipation, and other gastro disorders.

Therefore, if you want to feel a bit of back relief, you're generally transitioning the pain to your stomach, which could ultimately lead to even bigger issues, down the road.

As recently as March of 2015, however, researchers discovered a connection between cannabinoids and relief for back and neck pain. In the study, three different amounts of CBD oil was tested on some mice, all of which had a "condition" similar to that of back and neck pain. After they were given the various doses of CBD oil, the mice were given MRI scans to determine the damage within their bodies.

The mice that had the smaller doses of CBD oil had very little change. However, after fifteen days, the mice that had the higher CBD oil amounts actually showed decreased damage on a skeletal level: meaning that there are anti-degenerative effects when CBD oil is taken at a higher amount.

As a result, the scientists concluded that CBD oil could be utilized in the treatment of the cartilage discs in the back and neck, which could ultimately lead to decreased pain.

Thusly, there's a high probability that utilizing CBD oil to treat back and neck pain will result in decreased pain, and even regeneration of those lost cells. This could lead to better enjoyment of everyday life, management of chronic pain, and better sleep due to a decrease in pain.

A documented case: the benefits, her experience, and her life after using CBD oil every single day for pain relief.

The effects of CBD oil on everyday people— looking to pay their bills and live a normal life like you, are well-documented.

One woman in particular states that after doing quite a bit of heavy-lifting at her job, she began to strain her back. The back pain became persistent, forcing her to stay home and stop making money. She couldn't leave the house without assistance. She began to take heavy pain relievers, ones that zonked her out: making her dizzy, endlessly fatigued, and just foggy all the time. These pain relievers weren't natural; they were made in a lab. Due to these heavy side-effects, she turned to more medicinal and natural pain relief offered by CBD oil—something recommended to her by a friend who was using it to attempt to control her anxiety (something that she found success in).

After researching, the woman decided to begin taking approximately 3000 MG of CBD oil per month. She began by taking 30 MG per day and found that, with this new addition of pain relief, she didn't require any other pain medication throughout the day. Prior to CBD oil, she'd been forced to take pain medicine for her back at least twice per day.

Throughout the next few weeks, she made sure to take CBD oil every single morning, without forgetting. Within two hours of taking the 30 MG per day, she experienced no side effects and absolutely no back pain. She felt relaxed, finally finding the solace she so needed.

She also reported that, with CBD oil, her cognitive abilities were boosted, as was her overall mood. Therefore, the "side effects" of the "pain relief" involved an increase in quality of life, rather than ibuprofen side effects, like gastrointestinal duress.

Therefore, it is possible to completely replace your pain medications with CBD oil, eliminating the costs of lab-based products. It's well-documented and relief is waiting.

CHAPTER 4:
Rheumatoid Arthritis or Joint Pain and CBD Oil

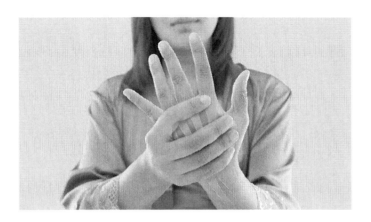

Rheumatoid arthritis is a silent, yet painful deformity that involves inflammation at the joints. This can cause pain along the ankles, wrists, fingers, and feet, and can even extend to swelling along inner body organs. The disease normally strikes between the ages of twenty-five and forty-five; however, it can even affect people as young as three or four.

What causes rheumatoid arthritis? Essentially, the issue strikes when pathogens are already wreaking havoc in normal tissue, causing inflammation. This inflammation then attacks the joints, spreading out to the bones and the surrounding cartilage. This leads to immobility on a joint level, and eventually deforms these joints, making them incredibly painful and unable to do normal tasks without crippling pain.

Many people exhibit different symptoms. It can involve continuous fatigue, pain and swelling in the joints, early-morning stiffness in the joints, weakness on a muscular level, and difficulties in sleeping.

If you suspect you have rheumatoid arthritis, you need to see your doctor as only an expert in the field can tell you for sure after an examination. However, knowing whether or not you have the disease, via this check-up, is incredibly clear, as rheumatoid arthritis makes itself known after only a short time.

Are You At Risk For Developing Rheumatoid Arthritis?

As mentioned, normally, rheumatoid arthritis makes itself known at the ages of between twenty-five and forty-five. Usually, the people who have the disease are female, over 75% of them. Furthermore, usually people who are diagnosed have a history of rheumatoid arthritis in their family, are obese, and are American Caucasians.

At this current point in medical therapy, physiotherapy involving cold, heat or other exercises that involve reduction of stiffness are generally utilized to decrease pain. Occupational therapy, as well as rest, are usually used, as are non-steroidal anti-inflammatory drugs, like ibuprofen. However, as mentioned in the previous chapter regarding back and neck pain, ibuprofen and other non-steroidal anti-inflammatory drugs can lead to other side effects, including inflammation in your inner organs and gastro-intestinal problems.

Treatment of Rheumatoid Arthritis with CBD Oil

According to several years of research, the utilization of CBD oil has been proven to improve rheumatoid arthritis, helping to reduce inflammation and pain of all types. This can further alleviate other joint-related inflammation, including inflammation from gout and osteoarthritis.

Throughout a period of five weeks during the year 2006, patients with rheumatoid arthritis used CBD oil every single day. This led to them reporting less pain and inflammation. Furthermore, when the rheumatoid arthritis was investigated via an MRI scanner, the inflammation was shown to have slowed in progress—meaning that, with CBD oil, rheumatoid arthritis won't have such a dramatic toll and can be slowed down. Therefore, the sentence of being unable to walk or move your hands in your later years? You can negate it.

In another study about CBD, published in the journal of Rheumatology by Chinese doctor Dr. Sheng-Ming Dai, it was found that something called CB2 receptors are found in incredibly high levels in the tissues around the joints of people with rheumatoid arthritis. When CBD oil is imbibed, this activates those pathways, which eliminates your brain's feeling of "pain" and leads to a decrease in inflammation. Therefore, according to experts in the field, patients who want a more natural answer to their arthritis should utilize CBD oil. It has none of the side effects of things like ibuprofen, which can cause gastro-intestinal duress. Furthermore, it may be more beneficial than other forms of therapy, including cold and heat.

The Best CBD Oils for Rheumatoid Arthritis

Green Roads World

The brand Green Roads has an incredible number and variety of CBD oils, which are all safe for consumption and also vaping. Regardless of what method you choose— vaping, taking by the mouth, through spray, etc.—you can opt for these products, which range between the prices of twenty-four dollars and sixty-four dollars, depending on strength. They offer high potency, meaning you'll get a good bang for your buck. Typically, Green Roads products affect you and alter your pain after about twenty or thirty minutes, and you generally don't have to take more than 30 MG per day.

CBDessence.net: Even if your pet is suffering from arthritis, this is safe for man or animal.

This line of products offer many different options for pain relief, including CBD-based products that involve vaping, capsule-taking, mix-in powders, pain relief for pets, oral tinctures, and other creams and gels. It can be delivered straight to your door, no matter what state you live in, and is safe for 30 to 35 MG of consumption per day.

Pure Kana

Pure Kana is one of the top manufacturers of CBD oil, across all reviews. Its extraction of CBD oil from the hemp plant is incredibly unique and precise, unlike other brands. With this technique, the company is able to create a CBD oil that's 99% pure. Its prices are fair, between forty-eight dollars and one hundred thirty-nine dollars, depending on what you get and what potency you want. It's safe to take in quantities of around 30 MG per day, and should ensure that you don't require another form of pain relief.

CHAPTER 5:
Fibromyalgia and CBD Oil

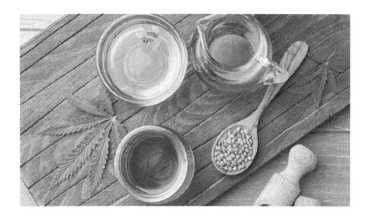

Fibromyalgia is a kind of chronic pain that leads to musculoskeletal irritation and a kind of overall, full-body pain, as well as cognitive disorders. According to doctors, there is absolutely no cure for this condition. Therefore, treatment for fibromyalgia requires a level of pain management—much like arthritis, back and neck pain.

Fibromyalgia was only recently said to be a legitimate disease, and therefore, not much is known about it. It's debilitating, and it's currently affecting the lives of millions of people. Here's what we do know about the horrors of this everyday disorder:

It was initially known as "yuppie flu," and was often referred to as a "syndrome," rather than an actual illness. It involves the many, many fibers in the body that "feel" pain, and then send the sensation of this pain back to the brain. This forces the body to experience pain all over the body, at the same time. Currently, fibromyalgia is the most frequent diagnosis, affecting women more often than men. At this time, stress is known to be a possible cause. This may be due to the fact that, over the previous twenty or thirty years, women have been subject to stressful problems more often than previously. Stress wreaks havoc on the body in ways doctors and scientists are still amazed by.

People who also suffer from fibromyalgia are also known to be more susceptible to other diseases, including irritable bowel syndrome, chronic fatigue syndrome, and even really bad migraines.

Therefore, what we do know about fibromyalgia involves the endocannabinoid system, which is the very system that receives signals from the body which then are translated as "pain." If you remember correctly, the very point of CBD oil is that it interferes with the endocannabinoid system, to your benefit, and then allows you to feel pain in a different way: often decreasing it in a dramatic fashion, leading to continued relief.

In essence, CBD oil binds to microglial cells in this endocannabinoid system, which in turn reduces the number of cytokines in the bloodstream. This reduces the amount of pain felt by people with fibromyalgia at a drastic level, due to the fact that microglial cells have been listed as the potential for inflammation and the dramatic fatigue found in fibromyalgia patients.

Could CBD Oil Be An Answer to Fibromyalgia?

When treating fibromyalgia as you would other pain-related problems, like migraines and headaches, you often turn to ibuprofen and other medicines with side-effects. Other treatments, including opioid pain medication, corticosteroids, and others, offer their other host of side effects and the potential for addiction.

However, CBD oil offers pain relief in just the same way as these other medicines and treatments, without the side effects. Due to the fact that little is known about fibromyalgia, all cases are different and should be treated accordingly. Thusly, just because another patient finds relief from fibromyalgia, doesn't mean you will, as well. However, due to the fact that it has little to no side effects, and can only help, CBD oil is therefore a valid choice.

A Poorly Regulated Endocannabinoid System?

It's also been purported that people with fibromyalgia have a deficient endocannabinoid system, meaning that it's unable to regulate the body's sleep, pain, appetite, mood, inflammation, and even sexual patterns. Since CBD oil has a direct effect on your endocannabinoid system, it could knock your body back into its normal patterns, leaving you the space to sleep, to reproduce, to experience only the pain you're meant to experience (the necessary, "ouch" kind that tells you not to hit your knee on a table again, etc.).

Best CBD Oil for Fibromyalgia

Despite the fact that fibromyalgia cannot be cured, CBD oil can be utilized to reduce discomfort and pain, with people sharing their success stores across the world. Individuals have reported they now experience a more positive brain space, each and every day, which pushes them to live their lives with more power and strength, not held back by the pain and low energy levels of their illness.

Here is a list of the best CBD oils for fibromyalgia, as reported by the millions of people who utilize it to treat their illness across the world.

Elixiol

Elixinol has an incredible reputation for being safe, with a high-potency and a good price. With Elixinol, you can find either unflavored or flavored CBD oil, with both mild and strong potency levels. The price ranges anywhere between thirty-nine dollars and two hundred and forty-nine dollars, depending on what you're looking for. It's safe to take at around 30 to 35 MG per dose, about twice a day.

CBD Pure

According to the website Marijuana Break, CBD oil from CBD Pure has three specializations, all with pure CBD extracts at different potency rates. They're continuously trying to master their formulas and ensuring that they're reaching toward a greater purity level. They have a 90-day happiness guarantee, meaning that if you're not happy after 90 days, you can actually get your money back. The products are completely organic, and actually all come from Denmark. A third-party lab always checks on the purity of the CBD oil, meaning that you're getting precisely what you paid for

CHAPTER 6:
Chronic Pain Management and CBD Oil

Everyone experiences pain. It's what you feel when you hurt your elbow, when you overdo it on the exercise machines at the gym, and when that space behind your eyes starts to feel achy and bad, due to your reading in poor light. However, when that pain crosses over into twelve weeks of consistent horror—it's considered chronic pain, and it can change and even ruin your life.

Unfortunately for sufferers of chronic pain, much of the answers in the medical universe are things that the body eventually grows accustomed to. The body needs higher and higher doses of medicine in order to feel better, and this ultimately leads to many bad side effects and risks against your gastrointestinal tract, as well as other parts of the body. Medicine can add up, expense-wise, and is ultimately just another path to destroying your body, rather than healing it in a natural way.

CBD oil is a potential answer to chronic pain, taking the place of ibuprofen and other pain relievers, with many people across the world turning to the natural CBD oil for relief.

What Causes Chronic Pain?

Chronic pain is usually caused from an injury. This can be a sprain in the ankle, a sprain in the back, or just a muscle sprain that occurs due to some kind of weakness. As a result of chronic pain, your body is often at the mercy of inability to sleep correctly, inability to eat, and other disturbances.

Unfortunately, little is known about eliminating chronic pain, beyond managing the pain itself.

Why Is CBD Oil Perfect for Managing Pain?

In a recent study, researchers decided to look at the way the brain processes pain in order to see how CBD oil can affect how your brain tells you if you're actually "feeling" it. Throughout the study, CBD was injected into rats, ultimately ensuring that the rats' brains and CBD came into contact for the sake of the study. The rats were further given a mechanical allodynia, which shows how they react to the feeling of pain. This would ensure the researchers could track how the CBD was flowing through the rats' endocannabinoid system.

After injecting the rats, it was shown that the feeling of pain fell away in the rats' pain receptors, meaning that CBD oil alters the way the rats' brains were communicating pain.

Furthermore, CBD oil was used orally to prove whether or not it diminished neuropathic or chronic inflammatory pain. In this study, the rats had suffered from something called a "sciatic nerve chronic constriction." This created a brain-based pain. The rats then received a treatment of CBD oil, orally, every single day.

After a single week of treatment, the pain in the rats was significantly decreased. Therefore, the scientists stated that the CBD oil could be a successful agent in reducing chronic pain.

CBD Oil and Chronic, Cancer-Related Pain

While CBD oil is an essential tool in treating chronic pain and injury-related pain, it can also be utilized for pain that is related to cancer. It's well-known that treatment of cancer is generally toxic, and can weaken the cells in your body. Treating this pain with more medicine, which can lead to further complications, isn't always an option, especially when these cancer patients are already taking a whole host of treatments.

Back in 2006, the US FDA approved CBD oil intake for cancer patients. Afterwards, cancer patients began to utilize CBD oil, looking to reduce adverse side effects. For all the reasons listed above, including CBD oil's effects on how the brain "reads" pain throughout the body, CBD oil is an incredible option for cancer pain relief. The only known side effects that were reported were:

brief dizziness, irritability, and fatigue.

CHAPTER 7:
Multiple Sclerosis and CBD Oil

Multiple sclerosis, otherwise known as MS, is a disease that, when diagnosed, will be with you the rest of your life. It affects everything from your spinal cord to your brain to the optic nerves in your eyes, and it ultimately alters your balance, the way you see the world, how you can control your muscles, and other bodily functions.

The effects of MS are incredibly different and far-reaching, depending on the person. Many people have only a few, small symptoms, and therefore don't even require treatment, while other people will struggle living out days of their lives.

Essentially, what happens when you have MS is this: your immune system attacks myelin, which is a fat substance that is meant to protect your nerve fibers. When you don't have this myelin, your nerves are damaged, which usually leads to scar tissue.

The symptoms of multiple sclerosis include: fatigue, inability or struggle with walking, sexual difficulties, tingling in the hands and feet, blurred vision, muscle spasms or just all around weakness, depression, and overall pain. The pain, on top of everything else? It can really take you out of the game. The symptoms for MS usually begin between the ages of 20 and 40, with most people's symptoms getting increasingly worse over time.

The cause of multiple sclerosis is unknown, unfortunately. Many things are linked to the disease, including genetics and smoking.

Treatment for MS is unfortunately lacking. This is leading many people who have been diagnosed to seek out CBD oil, which can assist with the following: It can reduce the amount of disturbances in sleep; it can reduce your daily spasms; it can reduce the pain that exists in your brain and other neural pathways; and it can reduce the spastic muscle motions.

According to many people who've experimented utilizing CBD oil for self-treatment, their symptoms have decreased at an incredible rate. One particular user reports that they purchased 500 mg of CBD oil in a two-ounce bottle and then began to utilize the tincture every single day, dotting a few drops of it beneath their tongue. They made sure they did this action every single day, regardless of how bad their symptoms were. They wanted to stay consistent, knowing that the side effects otherwise (just a bit of dizziness and occasional dry mouth) wouldn't affect their daily life. Also, they stated that sometimes, when they knew that, say, Wednesday would be overly difficult for them—physically and even mentally—they took a few extra drops of the tincture on Monday, just in preparation. When they did this every single day, they reported less tiredness, less spasms throughout their muscles, and, above all, less pain. Now that they've reportedly been using the tincture for the previous eight months, they've been able to have a more active and more vibrant lifestyle.

CHAPTER 8:
CBD Oil Brands, Packaging, and How Much to Pay

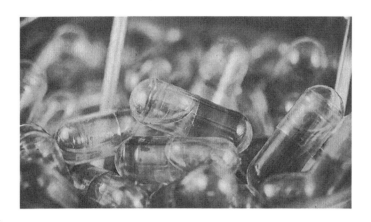

Purchasing CBD oil, knowing how to take it, and ensuring you aren't paying too much for a high quality product, can be rather difficult, especially as the industry continues to explode. Look to the following instructions to keep abreast of the current CBD oil landscape, along with our recommendations for best CBD oil products.

Different Versions of CBD Oil on the Market

Essentially, you can find three different, main versions of CBD oil on the market. There's Raw CBD Oil, Decarboxylated CBD Oil, and Filtered CBD Oil, otherwise known as the "gold" line.

Here's what you need to know about each type.

The Raw CBD Oil is known to be taken in its original format, without processing after it's taken directly from the plant. Therefore, the "raw" is taken literally. The oil contains chlorophyll and bits of the plant, which makes the color of Raw CBD oil a dark green or black. It's also thicker than other versions of CBD oil, as it hasn't been processed.

Generally, Raw CBD Oil is utilized by people who are wanting all the properties of a cannabis plant, rather than just what CBD oil can provide. It's the cheapest version of all the CBD oil varieties, and it is most often utilized for anxiety, depression, and insomnia. It's more on the mild side, as it's not as "pure" as other brands. This means that it's probably not going to handle big-time chronic pain as well as other strains.

Decarboxylated CBD Oil, on the other hand, is usually purchased by those CBD oil users wishing to bake up their own CBD oil edibles. These people are generally seeking out CBD oil to cure their depression, arthritis, headaches, migraines, anxieties, and other minor to moderate ailments.

But what does it mean that this CBD oil is "decarboxylated"? Essentially, when CBD oil is decarboxylated, the CBD oil has released a carbon atom from the inside of the CBD molecule. This morphs CBDA into CBD, which allows the molecule to fit better into the cell receptors in the endocannabinoid system (as mentioned, this is the process required to "interfere" with how your brain and body "feels" pain). This process makes decarboxylated CBD oil more powerful than Raw CBD Oil, as it works with the neural pathways in your body with more precision and power.

Therefore, decarboxylated CBD Oil is more powerful, meaning you have to take less of it to get the same benefits as Raw CBD Oil.

Filtered CBD Oil is the highest-priced of all the CBD oils, and it's the one that's most often purchased for medicinal use. People turn to it for anxiety, depression, and worse ailments—such as the ones listed in this book, like multiple sclerosis, arthritis, chronic pain, and others. It's decarboxylated and also filtered, meaning that the plant material and chlorophyll is completely eliminated, and the CBD oil is the only element that remains.

Best Brands of CBD Oil on the Market Right Now

The following brands of CBD oil are the absolute best on the market today, created in a lab specifically to supply a natural remedy to your current ailments.

Kat's Naturals

Kat's Naturals offers an incredible line of tinctures, with a 99.9% purity rate. They offer a number of tincture blends, with various flavors and "feelings," including "relax" and "heal." Their milligrams per ounce are impressive, with 250 milligrams of CBD oil per 10 milliliter bottle, 300 milligrams of CBD oil per 15 milliliter, and so on. Kat's also sells vape pens and even CBD oil products that your pets can take.

Populum

Populum is one of the most artistic CBD oil brands out there, with a gorgeous website and aesthetic. They offer three levels of their CBD oil stocks: the 250 milligrams basic level, the 500 milligrams signature level, and the 1000 milligrams advanced level. However, their prices are on the higher end of the spectrum, with a discount for people who subscribe.

Canabidol

This is a UK-based brand, offering multivitamins that contain CBD oils. This is best if you're more into taking CBD in a pill form. However, Canabidol also offers tinctures in 10 milliliter bottles, with various potencies, including 250 milligrams, 500 milligrams, and 1000 milligrams. Unlike Populum, Canabidol is on the cheaper end of the spectrum.

4 Corners Cannabis

This company is based in Colorado, and is known to offer top-of-the-line CBD products, straight from a Colorado farm. Their offerings include three tinctures, of 250 mg, 500 mg, and 1000 mg of strength. Because this is one of the best around, 4 Corners has prices on the higher end, with $200 for the higher potency.

Different CBD Oil Packaging

You might receive CBD oil a few different ways. These involve plastic jars, syringes, and silicone jars. Syringes are easier for the storage and the dispensing of CBD oil. However, if the CBD oil grows too cold within the syringe, it can be difficult to release the CBD oil from the syringe. A trick to fix this? Simply place the syringe in a bowl of warm water, or even wrap the syringe in a paper towel and heat it in the microwave for no more than five seconds.

Otherwise, silicone jars and plastic jars are generally used for Raw CBD Oil, which isn't something we recommend for the level of pain you're experiencing if you are reading this book.

Don't Get Blindsided: Know What You're Paying For

When purchasing CBD oil, it's essential to:

-Make sure the bottle lists the percentage of CBD oil within the bottle.
-Make sure that the CBD oil has been tested in a third-party laboratory.

-Calculate how much you're paying per milligram of CBD oil, to ensure you're not being taken advantage of.

When shopping for anything else, be it groceries or even medicine, it's usually easy to compare how much everything costs and then decide on which brand to buy. We normally compare the price to the weight or volume of whatever we're buying and then make a calculated decision. However, calculating the price of your CBD is a bit more difficult, when faced with big bottles versus smaller bottles.

The question is: Which will give you a bigger bang for your buck, in terms of oil?

You can only do this if you know the percentage of CBD oil or amount of milligrams of CBD oil within the bottle you wish to purchase.

From this, you can do a bit of calculation to ensure you're getting a good price on each milligram of CBD oil. This ensures the oil isn't too "watered down," in a sense. This also ensures you know how many milligrams you're taking when you self-medicate. You don't want to take it blindly, after all. Too much is too much, and too little will have no effect at all.

For example, let's say you're purchasing a 20 ml bottle of oil, which is said to contain 600 mg of CBD oil. Let's say the bottle costs ninety-nine dollars. To work out how much the price per milligram is, simply divide $99 by the number of milligrams of CBD: 600. In this case, you'll find that you're paying $0.165 per milligram of CBD oil.

Note that bigger bottles generally set you up for failure. They advertise themselves as big bottles at lower prices. However, if the big bottle doesn't list the percentage of CBD oil within it, then it's probably taking advantage of you and not offering much CBD oil.

CHAPTER 9:
CBD Oil Dosing and How to Take It

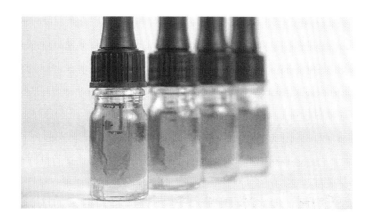

How Much of the CBD Oil Should You Take Per Day?

According to several CBD oil specialists, the amount of CBD oil you should take per day depends on you, your body size, and your level of pain.

Therefore, there's no direct scientific information that can point to the exact amount of CBD oil you should be taking. It's a natural remedy, and that's just how these things work. However, according to the FDA, CBD oil is meant to be treated much as you would food. Therefore, it comes with a label calling out the "serving size." This serving size is probably incorrect for your usages, meaning that you'll have to experiment with CBD intake to arrive at how much you should take to alleviate pain.

Many brands, for example, state that 10 drops are an appropriate serving size, along with how many milligrams of CBD oil are contained in those 10 drops. Let's say that, in this brand, 10 drops of CBD oil equates to only 5 mg of CBD oil. However, perhaps you've discovered—through trial and error, as well as the following tools, that you require at least 10 mg per day, or per usage. This means you'll need at least 20 droplets of this particular brand, which is double what the brand calls the "serving size." Therefore, that serving size is not to be trusted.

As mentioned, the amount of CBD oil you should take per day depends on your weight and how serious your condition is. If you're bigger, you should take in more CBD oil. If you're in more pain, you should take more CBD oil. It sounds simple. But here's a way to keep things in line.

For Minor Pain, Here's What You Should Take:

Let's say your baby is experiencing minor pain and is under 25 pounds. The starting amount of CBD oil should be no more than 4.5 mg. If your child is between 26 and 45 pounds, and is experiencing minor pain, start at around 6 mg of CBD oil. If your child is between 46 and 85 pounds, try 9 mg of CBD oil. If you're between 86 and 150 pounds, try 12 mg of CBD oil. Between 151 and 240 pounds, try 18 mg of CBD oil. And if you're over 240 pounds, opt for 22.5 mg of CBD oil.

For Moderate Amounts of Pain, Here's What You Should Take:

Below 25 pounds, take 6 mg of CBD oil. Between 26 pounds and 45 pounds, try 9 mg. Between 46 and 85 pounds, take 12 mg of CBD oil. Between 86 pounds and 150 pounds, take 15 mg of CBD oil. Between 151 and 240 pounds, take 22.5 mg of CBD oil. Over 240 pounds, take 30 mg of CBD oil.

For Severe Amounts of Pain, Here's What You Should Take:

Below 25 pounds, take 9 mg of CBD oil. Between 26 pounds and 45 pounds, take 12 mg. Between 46 and 85 pounds, take 15 mg of CBD oil. Between 86 and 150 pounds, take

19 mg. Between 151 pounds and 240 pounds, take 27 mg. Over 240 pounds, try 45 mg of CBD oil.

Know that you should experiment with what is listed above. These are good "jumping off points." If you don't feel any change at all, you can move up with your intake, knowing that you really can't take too much. You really can't eat too much broccoli, for example; but at a certain point, it probably isn't going to give you all the benefits it can, as your body can only handle so much at once.

Therefore, the amount of mg per person is generally between 4 and 30 mg per day, depending on their size and the severity of their situation. If you have severe back pain and weigh between 86 and 150 pounds, then it's recommended you start out taking 19 mg. If you're suffering from anxiety and weigh between this range, then it's recommended you take between 12 mg and 15 mg the first time.

When you're first experimenting with CBD oil, it's important to experiment with your dosage amounts. It's recommended that you take your given dosage amount once in the morning AND once in the evening. You should take it twice during the first four days in order to build up the CBD oil in your system. After these first four days, simply drop down to once per day. At this point, your body will be reacting to CBD oil—alerting you to whether or not you need those double doses or can handle just one.

Top Ways to Take CBD Oil

You can take CBD oil in a variety of ways, including: topically, on your skin; as a spray; as a capsule; as a tincture; or as a concentrate.

CBD Oil as a Concentrate

When you take your CBD oil as a concentrate, you're ensuring you get the highest dose. It has more than ten times the concentration than any of the other ways of taking CBD oil, and is considered more potent, more able to tackle your pain relief—and thus, something to be wary of, as researchers recommend you don't take more than 30 or 35 mg per day.

The things you might not like about CBD oil as a concentrate? It doesn't come in any other flavors, which means it offers nothing but the "natural flavor," which takes a bit of getting used to. Plus, concentrate always comes in a syringe, or a needle, which means it can be a bit scary in the initial days of usage.

To use this concentrate, simply bring the tip of the needle beneath your tongue or along the inside of your cheeks and eject the concentrate along the inner lining. Don't swallow the stuff. Rather, just allow it to be ingested slowly, over time.

This will give you the most instantaneous pain relief, and, alongside tinctures, is generally recommended.

CBD Oil as a Capsule

Taking a simple pill of CBD oil is definitely the easiest way of getting the medicinal properties, however not always the most potent. Each capsule of CBD oil contains between 10 and 25 mg of CBD oil, which allows you to keep track of how much CBD oil you're taking each time—without having to calculate it or measure it out.

The only issue is that sometimes, you might want to increase your CBD oil intake per day. But with a pill, you must double your intake, rather than doing it gradually.

CBD Oil as a Tincture

Much like concentrate, CBD oil tinctures are incredibly pure. Unlike concentrates, tinctures offer a bit of flair and flavor, which can makes them a bit more enjoyable.

To do this, simply dot a few droplets of the tincture's CBD oil beneath your tongue. Don't swallow. Instead, allow it to gradually fall down your throat and seep into your system.

CBD Oil Used Topically

CBD oil is utilized in topical creams and salves, which offer incredible skin benefits, can be anti-psoriasis, anti-inflammation, anti-acne, anti-wrinkles, and can even assist with managing the pain caused by arthritis. However, when purchasing CBD oil as a cream, it's essential to buy ones that use nano technology or "micellization," which makes sure that the CBD oil cream can enter the skin, rather than staying on top of it and gradually coming off.

CBD Oil Taken as a Spray

The concentration of most CBD oil sprays is incredibly low, making this the least recommended way to take CBD oil. Usually, each spray carries between 1 mg and 3 mg of CBD oil, which is nothing compared to that 25 mg pill. Each time you spray, it's difficult to measure out how much you're taking, as well. The range of measurement could be very off.

CBD Oil Breathed In Through a Vape

According to some people who use CBD oil religiously, vaping—or inhaling—CBD oil lends a more "even" intake of CBD oil. This is because, when you ingest anything, it's impossible to know how quickly it's absorbed into your system, depending on when you're taking it throughout your eating schedule.

To smoke CBD oil, you must buy a vaporizer or an e-cigarette. You'll insert the oil into the device, turn on the device, and then smoke the device the way you might a cigarette or a cigar. Then, blow out the smoke.

When Does CBD Oil Kick In?

When you take enough for your system (given the information in this paragraph), CBD oil shouldn't taken more than twenty or thirty minutes to kick in. Most people can't "feel" it taking over, since it doesn't give you a high—

like it's brother, THC. Usually you can't really notice the subtle feeling of it until you grow more accustomed to it over the span of several days.

CHAPTER 10:
CBD Oil Recipes to Manage Everyday Pain

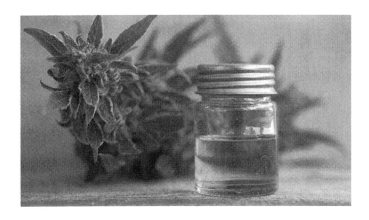

While you can purchase topical creams that already contain CBD oil, sometimes it's nice—and cheaper—to just make the produces at home with the CBD oil you already have. This way, you can personalize the smells, make just enough for the week, and cut down on plastic and other packaging on your road to better health and mindfulness.

In the first recipe, I'll walk you through how to make your own CBD oil from dried cannabis—something you don't have to do if you're already buying CBD oil yourself (but certainly something that's beneficial to know).

Simple CBD Salve

Ingredients:
1/3 cup jojoba oil
1 1/3 cups coconut oil
9 grams dried cannabis, ground
1/3 cup beeswax
10 drops lavender essential oil

1 cup aloe vera
3 tbsp. cocoa butter

Extra Items Required:
1 cheesecloth
1 baking sheet
1 jar

Directions:
First, preheat your oven to 240 degrees Fahrenheit. Spread out the cannabis on the baking sheet, after grinding it. When the oven is preheated, add the baking sheet to the oven and allow it to decarboxylate for 30 minutes. (Remember, this means that the CBD will be more "pure" and better at interacting with your body's neural receptors).

While the cannabis decarboxylates, add the coconut oil and jojoba oil to a saucepan. Heat over low heat, stirring constantly.

After the cannabis is done baking, remove it from the oven and add it to the coconut oil mixture. Keep cooking at low heat, stirring all the time for 25 minutes. If you don't stir continuously at a very low heat, the cannabis might burn—which isn't what you want.

After stirring, remove the mixture from the heat and pour it through a cheesecloth, directly into a storage jar.

Next, add the beeswax to the saucepan and heat it until it's completely melted. As the wax melts, add the coconut oil back into the saucepan. Stir well, and add the essential oils at this time.

After mixing together the ingredients, remove the mixture from the heat and add the cocoa butter and the Aloe Vera gel. Stir well.

Then, store the mixture in the jar. Use the salve on your aches and pains as needed.

Super Intense Moisturizing Arthritis and Neck Pain Lotion

Ingredients:

20 mg CBD oil
1 1/2 tsp. grated beeswax
2 tsp. Shea butter
12 drops lavender essential oil

Directions:

First, place the Shea better and the beeswax in a bowl that can be microwaved, and heat it in the microwave for one minute on medium-high. Afterwards, add the CBD oil and the essential oils. Stir well, and pour the mixture into a plastic container so that it can set.

Once it's hardened, apply the moisturizer on your muscles, your skin, or the joints of your hands and feet for relief.

Stiff Neck and Back Oil

Ingredients:
50 mg CBD oil
10 drops eucalyptus essential oil
2 tbsp. olive oil

Directions:
Stir together the ingredients and store them together in a small squeeze bottle. Add the massage oil over your sore hands, feet, muscles, shoulders, or neck, any time you feel the aches and pains. Allow the mixture to absorb through your skin first, before putting on clothing.

Calming Body Butter

Ingredients:
15 drops peppermint essential oil
1/2 cup cocoa butter
1/3 cup magnesium oil
1/3 cup coconut oil
40 mg CBD oil

Directions:
First, add the cocoa butter and the coconut oil to a saucepan and heat over medium heat. Allow them to melt together, stirring frequently, before removing it from the heat.

At this time, add the magnesium oil, along with the peppermint essential oils. Then, add the CBD oil and stir well. Allow the mixture to cool.

When the mixture cools, whip the mixture using a whisk or a hand mixer, creating a fluffy and light texture. Add the CBD butter to a container and apply any time you feel aches and pains.

30145880R00043

Printed in Poland
by Amazon Fulfillment
Poland Sp. z o.o., Wrocław